Fasting:a way of being fit

David Rolland

DEDICATION

I dedicate this book to God almighty for his Mercy and grace in my life. I also dedicate this book to my late dad who is my motivator and my hero

CONTENTS

ACKNOWLEDGMENTS

I want to acknowledge my brother for helping me out in the publishing of this book. He is truly a wise person and I thank God for him.
I also want to acknowledge my mother for the advice she has been giving me throughout this period.

1. WHAT IS FASTING

Fasting, according to the dictionary," is the abstinence from food."

It can as well be applied to the abstinence of things like phones, social media, meat Etc.

It is one of the ways that people find useful in maintaining weight, being fit, and staying healthy.

Someone in one of the social media handles asked one of the richest men in the world by **name of Elon musk, "What is his secret of being fit?"**

He said it was fasting.

Fasting has helped many people in the world today to realize their true selves and help them to improve their health conditions and vice versa.

Fasting can also be seen as the ability to not eat for some time which might be for 2 days or more to achieve a particular goal

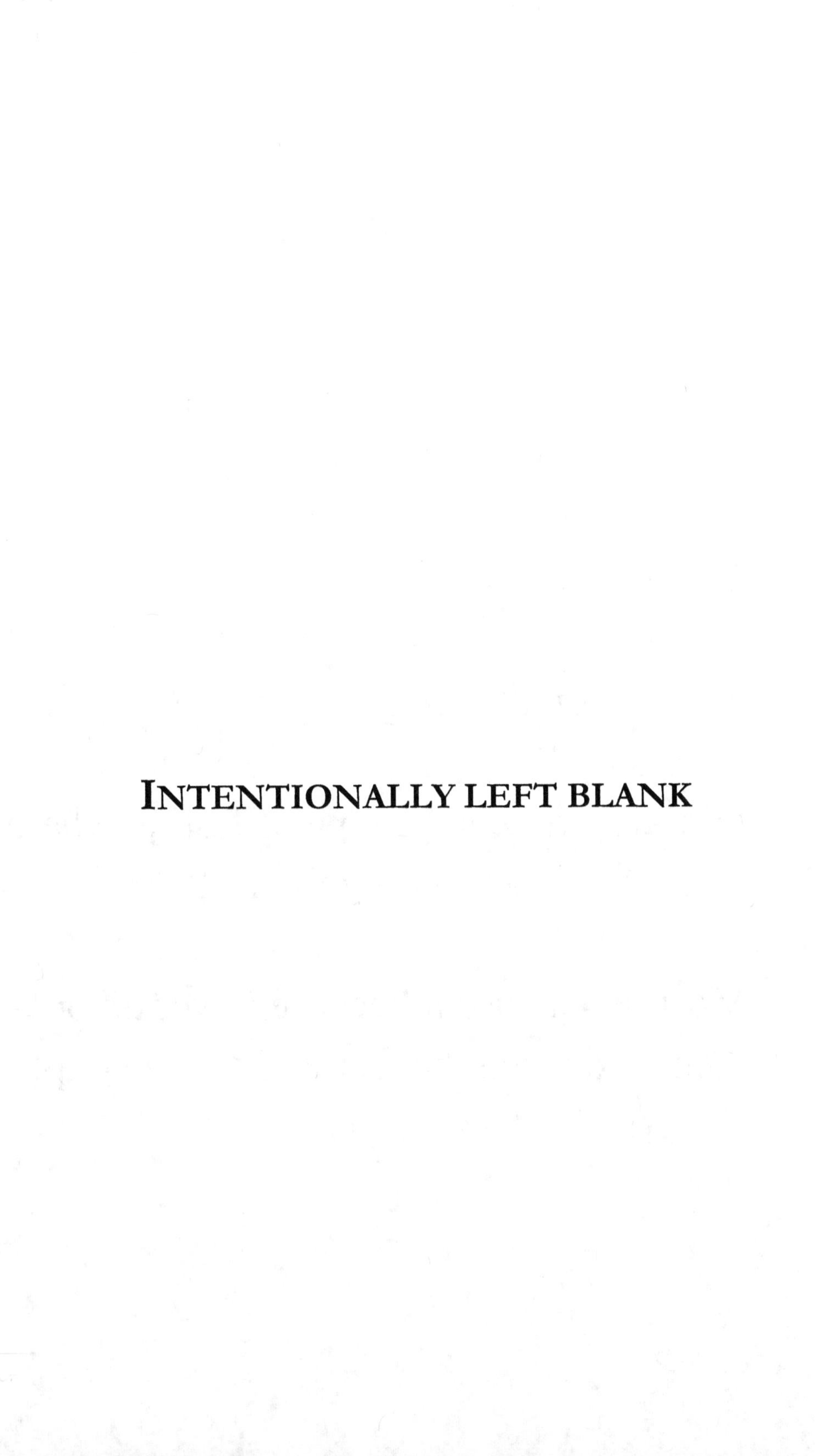

INTENTIONALLY LEFT BLANK

2. Types of Fasting

They are different types of fasting but I am mainly going to focus on two:
1. Partial fasting
2. Dry fasting

Partial fasting

Partial fasting is the type of fasting where you drink water during the fast.

Most people use it because it works for them and when the fast will take a couple of days (3-7days).

It is advisable to take water during that fast because it helps to wash your bowels and makes you hydrated at all times.

One thing with partial fasting is that it trains you to start the real deal which is Dry fasting.

Dry fasting

Dry fasting is a type of fasting where the person does not take anything and goes about his daily business.

Some people do this type of fasting for two days.

It is one of the best but it is demanding.

That is why I would advise you to start from partial fasting and graduate to dry fasting.

INTENTIONALLY LEFT BLANK

3. How to do fasting properly?

This is not a big deal because anyone can do fasting.

I would advise if the person starts from 12 am to 12 pm for a start or 6 pm.

During this period, the person should not drink water if it will last for a day.

But if it is going to last for days, he should drink water during the fast to wash the bowels.

I would also advise him to read Christian books like the bible or a Christian literature
during the fast.

I know that you are fasting to be fit but this is one thing you don't know about fasting.

The thing is that it will make you discover more about yourself which helps if you ask me.

You can also pray during that period of fasting and ask God what you want him to do for you.

You can equally table the matter of your weight to him(Jesus).

One of the ways to lose weight is to stop eating late-night food.

Do not eat beyond 6 pm if you want to lose weight and be fit mentally, physically, and emotionally.

It is also advisable to sleep early and have a good night's sleep of 6hrs.

INTENTIONALLY LEFT BLANK

4. How does fasting help in the physical?

1. It helps you to be fit

2. It helps you to lose weight

3. It Improves your health status

4. It makes you feel relieved of anything you are passing through

5. It gives you the ability to conquer temptation

INTENTIONALLY LEFT BLANK

5. Advantages of fasting

According to an article by Rachel link :

1. It promotes blood sugar control by reducing insulin resistance.

2. AIDS WEIGHT LOSS BY LIMITING CALORIE INTAKE

3. IT INCREASES GROWTH HORMONE SECRETION AND MUSCLE STRENGTH.

4. IT COULD DELAY AGING.

5. IT ALSO INCREASES THE LONGEVITY OF HUMANS

INTENTIONALLY LEFT BLANK

6. How does fasting help in the physical?

1. It helps you to be fit

2. It helps you to lose weight

3. It Improves your health status

Spiritual life?

1. It makes you discover yourself

2. Your inner spirit grows because you are feeding it with the words from the Bible and starving the flesh/grows your spirit.

3. It gives you the ability to conquer temptation

INTENTIONALLY LEFT BLANK

7. What to fast from?

1. Food: We ought to fast from food because it is the primary thing to fast from Food like calories sugar, gluten, etc

This will go a long way in helping you to grow your spirit.

When we are fasting for that day, we should, first of all, eat fruits before eating any other thing.

The fruit has a way of helping the body immediately after fasting.

2. Phone:Nowadays our phone is now a distraction to us.

We can't do without our phones and that is why we should fast from them.

It is taking most of our time and which is not good.

We should have some days we fast from our phone to do other things etc

3. Social media:This is one of the most important forms of communication we have in the world today.

We have different social media platforms which you all are acquainted with such as

Facebook, Instagram, Twitter, Whatsapp
Etc

We have a variety of communication
platforms thanks to the people that
invented them.

This is one of the reasons we should fast
from it in a day because it has now
become part of our life.

their

8. Importance of Fasting

1. It makes you live long

2. It makes you lose weight

3. It makes you achieve the main thing
in this book because we all want to be fit.

It normally deals with not eating but
drinking water.

When one does not eat for some time,
one becomes fit too.

When fasting is done well, the person becomes better than before.

4. It makes your blood pressure to be normal or improves your health:

When one fast, he stays away from food especially those that have high cholesterol.

Cholesterol has a way of triggering or increasing blood pressure in humans.

Fasting helps to reduce that in the life of a person.

INTENTIONALLY LEFT BLANK

9. Benefits of Fasting

1. it helps to conquer temptation:When you fast, it gives you the ability to conquer temptation.

2. It helps your inner spirit to be strong which will make you overcome any temptation that will come your way.

3. It will make you not fall into something that you will regret afterward.

4. It helps you to have self-control:Fasting can help you to have self-control because for that period your flesh

is weak and you are controlling your body not to eat much.

5. It will make you know some certain things you have to stop doing.

6. It makes you lose weight:This is the one that most of you like. Yes, fasting will make you lose weight.

It has made many people lose weight because they have not been eating well.

The thing behind it is that fasting will equally make you look better than before and fit.

8. It makes you discover yourself:As you fast from food and meditate on God's Word(the Bible) the life of Christ starts forming in you.

Your own life starts to reflect in your eyes and you will know where you are getting it all wrong.

You start making amends in your life and you see yourself becoming the best of yourself

9. It makes you live long:One of the benefits of fasting is that it makes you live longer because you have decided to fast from food which is essential for living to grow your spirit man.

Fasting enables you to go on with your daily activities without eating food but drinking water only.

Water is very essential for living and it washes your bowels alongside your kidneys.

NB:If you are going to end your fasting in a day let us say by 6 pm, eat fruit first before anything.

Don't rush into drinking water if it is dry fasting because of some activities that will be taking place in the stomach due to that you have not drank water during the day.

After eating those fruits then you can proceed to drink water and then eat.

ABOUT THE AUTHOR

David Rolland is an author that is interested in adding value to people's lives by writing it down in a book. He likes to write quality books that will help the reader at all times or keep him company.